SLOW DOWN
TO HEAL
AND
TRULY LIVE

TWENTY-ONE BIBLE-BACKED PRACTICES
TO NURTURE YOUR MIND, BODY, AND SPIRIT

PATRICIA MCNAMARA

WESTBOW
PRESS®
A DIVISION OF THOMAS NELSON
& ZONDERVAN

Disclaimer: The content in Slow Down to Heal and Truly Live is for informational and inspirational purposes only and is not a substitute for professional medical, psychological, or spiritual advice. Always consult with a qualified professional regarding any health concerns. The author and publisher are not liable for any outcomes related to the application of information in this book. Readers should engage with the practices thoughtfully and choose what aligns with their well-being and beliefs.

WestBow Press books may be ordered through booksellers or by contacting:

WestBow Press
A Division of Thomas Nelson & Zondervan
1663 Liberty Drive
Bloomington, IN 47403
www.westbowpress.com
844-714-3454

Scripture quotations are taken from the Holy Bible, NEW INTERNATIONAL VERSION®, NIV® Copyright © 1973, 1978, 1984, 2011 by Biblica, Inc.® Used by permission. All rights reserved worldwide.

ISBN: 979-8-3850-3732-2 (sc)
ISBN: 979-8-3850-3733-9 (hc)
ISBN: 979-8-3850-3734-6 (e)

Library of Congress Control Number: 2024923251

Print information available on the last page.

WestBow Press rev. date: 11/14/2024

To the One with endless patience, who has never given up on me. Thank You for picking me up time and time again and for showing me that I needed to slow down to heal and find my purpose. My hope is this devotional will bring You glory and serve Your kingdom well.

Thanks also to my husband and kids for believing in me and supporting me with this project. You bring me so much joy, and I love being your wife and mother!

And a special shout-out to my sister, Jane. She has been my Christian mentor for many years and encouraged me to pursue this project.

CONTENTS

PREFACE

After practicing in the health and wellness space for over five years as a nutritional therapy practitioner, I realized that many of my clients struggled with true healing even when they were doing "all the right things." Diet had been dialed in, and movement was prioritized. The missing link was the clients' ability to slow down and prioritize practices that nurture the mind, body, and spirit. After years of the do, do, do and go, go, go mentality, the body whispers and then perhaps eventually screams for reprieve, and symptoms start to appear.

These symptoms vary from person to person, but often include fatigue, insomnia, digestive complaints, and hormonal imbalances. This can eventually lead to anxiety and depression, autoimmune disease, high blood pressure, weight gain, and chronic diseases like diabetes and heart disease.

God knows the importance of slowing down and prioritizes it in His word. In Luke 5:15–16 we hear of Jesus often withdrawing to pray and rest, even when the sick and lost needed Him. He gives the perfect example of how we cannot give from an empty cup, and how important it is to care for ourselves—both to feel our best and to be useful in His Kingdom.

I learned the hard way how important slowing down and caring for our bodies is to health and well-being. As a recovering people-pleasing, type A personality, I defined my worth based on what I was completing and how I was contributing. This led to frequently putting others first at the expense of my own health. After the sudden loss of my mother and unrelenting health issues of my own, God revealed to me it was necessary to slow down and take time to care for my mind, body, and spirit.

What does it take to live a healthy and fulfilling life? God has all the answers and more in His special gift to us, the Bible. This devotion combines insights from God's word with common practices you can adopt to nurture your mind, body, and spirit. It will explain why the practices are beneficial to health and well-being, offer tips to help you get started, give you a place to reflect, and recommend action steps to motivate you.

With a healthier mind, body, and spirit we are better equipped to serve the Lord and others, which is our ultimate purpose here on earth.

INTRODUCTION

I was lying on my yoga mat, preparing to dig into my first writing session for this devotional. I was optimistic that I would hear from God to provide direction. After all, I had taken a couple minutes out of my oh-so-busy life to halfway listen for Him. I shook my head, realizing God deserves so much more than my halfhearted attention. But that requires slowing down. Why is it so hard for me to slow down, I wondered?

As I rolled up to head to the computer, I noticed my monstera plant needed watering. There were a couple of new leaves (babies as my friend Kimberly would say) that were almost dried up. My first instinct was that I should run and grab some water, even though I had promised God and myself that I would start at ten o'clock with no interruptions, no excuses.

A few minutes earlier, as I was rushing from my walk to my time working on this project, several other chores called for attention: watering the hanging baskets, cleaning the pool shark so that it could get a head start cleaning for the day, flipping a load of laundry. The list goes on and on. And honestly, any other day I would have pushed off the project to get these things done. You see, I am very good at doing and not very good at being.

We type A overachievers often have a really hard time in stillness. For me it took almost fifty-four years to realize worth is not based on work and busyness; our worth is determined by the fact that we are children of God. He created us and that is what makes us valuable. Do newborn babies provide any value (other than being absolutely adorable and cuddly)? No, yet we would never say that they are worthless because they don't contribute or get everything done on their to-do list.

My intention with *Slow Down to Heal and Truly Live* is to remind us that we are children of God who were created "to be" just as much as "to do." When we overlook our need for rest and nurturing, we burn out, we get sick or discouraged, and we quite possibly miss God's purpose for us in this life.

That certainly was the case for me. Voted most likely to succeed by my high school classmates, I had something to prove. My to-do list was never far from sight or mind. I graduated summa cum laude from college and started my career in investment banking. The next big step was marriage and motherhood. After several years in the finance world, I transitioned to becoming a stay-at-home mom. It's really hard to validate your worth in this role, so I went to town reading and researching what it took to be the "best mom." While I obviously fell short, I kept pushing to be the best I could be. I was stressed over creating the perfect home, yard, and life for my family.

Obsessing over my family's health concerns eventually led to me pursuing a career in nutrition and functional health. It was in this role that God spoke to me. If I wanted to heal and live the life He had planned for me, it was time to start practicing what I preach to my clients. I needed to slow down and prioritize practices that nurtured my body, not run it into the ground. A healthier me would ultimately allow me to help more people and hopefully bring them closer to God in the process.

I chose twenty-one Bible-backed practices because the number twenty-one in the Bible symbolizes divine completion and spiritual maturity. It represents the perfect blend of seven (God's creation) and three (the Trinity), signifying a higher level of completeness. The number twenty-one also marks the end of significant spiritual journeys, making it a powerful number that reflects a full, mature, and spiritually complete approach to health.

While I have not perfected all these practices (perfection is not the goal), I am healthier, happier, and better equipped to serve God and others. My hope is that you, too, will prioritize these practices and enjoy better health and a closer relationship with our Lord and Savior.

These twenty-one Bible-backed practices are not meant to overwhelm you, but rather to support you on your healing and growing journey. Utilize as many or as few as your life stage allows. There will always be seasons of busyness where we need to give ourselves grace and prioritize just a few of the practices.

I recommend taking something away versus adding one more thing to do; we are trying to slow down, after all! Rather than feeling like you need to add more to your already full plate, consider removing something that doesn't necessarily serve you—like less TV, less time on your phone, or fewer unnecessary obligations.

The goal is to create space for these practices, allowing you to reconnect with what truly matters—your relationship with God and your well-being. By simplifying your life, you'll open up room for healing, peace, and spiritual growth.

REST AND SELF-CARE

Then, because so many people were coming
and going that they did not even have a chance
to eat, he said to them, "Come with me by
yourselves to a quiet place and get some rest."
—Mark 6:31

PROPER REST ESCAPED me for most of my adult years. I held the belief that if you weren't busy doing something, you were lazy or wasting time. When I did rest (I love naps), I felt it needed to be justified. You see, there were New Year's resolutions and goals to achieve, and people to impress. Kids to raise, businesses to build, volunteering to be done, and a hardworking farm-girl reputation to uphold.

It took working with sick clients (almost always type A overachievers like yours truly) and getting sick myself to realize that rest is necessary and good. You can be doing all the right things (diet, exercise, biohacking), but if you are not supporting your body with rest, your health will eventually suffer.

Jesus rested, even when there were crowds of people who needed Him. God also showed the importance of rest when He rested on the seventh day of creation.

1

How do we rest more and practice self-care? Like many of the practices I recommend, this will require you to slow down. It's OK to say no and set boundaries.

Sundays are my days to rest (that doesn't mean I don't rest on other days as well). You can sometimes find me in my bed taking a nap, taking an Epsom salt bath, hanging in the hammock, or reading on the porch. Many days, I do a "mental reboot nap." I lie down for about thirty minutes to recharge my battery. It's like a mini reset, and I find myself much more productive afterward.

I'm also a huge fan of bodywork. I regularly see my chiropractor and massage therapist. My husband would often tease me about how for years I would justify my massage (because self-care is selfish, right?). When I would speak of this self-care practice, I made sure everyone knew it was a "deep-tissue massage" necessary to prevent my back from acting up. The truth is self-care is not a luxury; it is a necessity. I now feel proud instead of guilty for caring for the temple God entrusted to me. So go ahead and schedule that massage, spa day, or even just a nice relaxing bath or whatever self-care practice brings you joy and rest! When we take care of ourselves, we have more to give to others.

Why are rest and self-care necessary and beneficial to the mind, body, and spirit?

- Rest and self-care slow the heart rate and lower blood pressure.
- They reduce stress hormones and chronic stress.
- They promote calm and save energy.
- They reduce the risk of heart disease.
- They enhance digestion and alleviate stress-related issues.

- They regulate breathing and prevent hyperventilation.
- They relax muscles and reduce tension.
- They reduce pain and release natural painkillers.
- They improve blood sugar control and support diabetes management.
- They boost the immune system and enhance infection resistance.
- They heal the body and promote mental health.
- They increase productivity and creativity.
- They enhance decision-making and problem-solving skills.

Tip

Perhaps your budget doesn't allow for things like massages and spa days. Let your loved ones know that if they are looking for gift ideas, you would love a spa day or massage. You can also have a spa day at home—a nice relaxing Epsom salt bath or a DIY facial. Or consider trading off with a spouse or friend who could also benefit from a massage.

Prayer

Father, Son, and Holy Spirit, thank You for the gift of rest. With so many things vying for my attention, help me to remember that rest is necessary and good. Without it, my health and relationships suffer, including my relationship with You. Thanks also for Your example of rest in the Bible. If Jesus made it a priority, I can trust that it is important for me as well.

Reflection

If God (who is all-knowing) prioritizes rest, what is holding me back from giving my body the self-care and rest it requires?

....

....

....

....

....

....

....

....

....

....

Action Step

Schedule a facial, massage, or any other self-care practice that you enjoy.

Self-care is not selfish. You cannot
serve from an empty vessel.
—Eleanor Brownn

MOVEMENT/EXERCISE

Don't you know that you yourselves are God's
temple and that God's Spirit dwells in your midst?
—1 Corinthians 3:16

MOVEMENT IS ESSENTIAL in caring for ourselves—the temple where the Holy Spirit dwells. Exercise has always been a big part of my life, but for most of that time for the wrong reasons. I didn't work out to care for the temple God had blessed me with but rather because I thought I needed to lose weight and look good. I didn't realize until a few years ago just how much joy I experience walking the roads in our valley, how close to God I feel as I hike, and how important strength training is for a midlife woman's health (it's way more than just weight related). I finally switched my focus from how movement affects my outside to how it affects where the Spirit dwells.

Although exercise is beneficial, it's important not to overdo it, as excessive strain on the body can elevate cortisol levels and lead to added stress. Cortisol is a necessary hormone but can have negative health consequences when it is too high (or too low). I often see over-exercising hinder healing, especially in my type-A clients.

Gentle movement, such as walking, is a great place to start. Is it beneficial to engage in other activities like strength training, biking, swimming, and an occasional run? Absolutely. Just be conscious of stress that could arise from these activities. If you are undergoing a stressful time in your life, I would recommend gentle movement and taking a break from or cutting back on exercises like HIIT and long steady cardio.

Why is movement necessary and beneficial to the mind, body, and spirit?

- Movement helps you maintain independence and your physical abilities.
- It reduces health risks and the need for medical visits.
- It boosts energy and reduces fatigue.
- It improves balance and lowers the risk of falls.
- It manages and prevents diseases like heart disease and diabetes.
- It enhances sleep quality.
- It reduces stress and anxiety.
- It supports healthy weight management.
- It controls blood pressure.
- It improves cognitive functions like focus and planning.
- It enhances emotional well-being and reduces depression.
- It boosts mood and feelings of empowerment.

Tip

Schedule some form of movement and just start. Tell yourself you are going for ten minutes, and after ten minutes, you will probably feel like going longer. If not, ten minutes is better than nothing! Also, look at movement/exercise as something you get to do instead of having to do. Be grateful for your body and have realistic expectations. Slow and steady wins the race.

Prayer

Father in heaven, I'm so incredibly grateful for the body You have blessed me with; however, I have not always honored it. Forgive me for those times. Help me to accept my body for what it is (and isn't) and to prioritize movement each and every day.

Reflection

Take an inventory of your current exercise regime. Ask yourself, *Am I overtraining or too sedentary? What changes will I commit to in order to allow at least some gentle movement each day?*

....
....
....
....
....
....
....
....
....
....
....
....
....
....
....

Action Step ───────────────────────

If you are struggling with not enough movement, schedule a ten-minute walk in the next couple of days.

If you are perhaps pushing too hard when it comes to movement, can you swap a strenuous workout with a walk or yoga session?

> Walking is man's best medicine.
> —Hippocrates

MORNING SUNLIGHT

Light is sweet, and it pleases the eyes to see the sun.
—Ecclesiastes 11:7

NOTHING INVIGORATES ME more than feeling sunshine
on my face. It's like a great big hug from God. There are many
mornings during my quiet time with God when I can feel the
sun getting brighter and warmer on my body. I feel like God is
letting me know He is pleased and loves me.

My morning walks with my dog Maize are always better
when the sun peeks through the trees. It's a constant reminder
that He is the sun, and I am the moon. Although I have no light
of my own, I can reflect Him.

Why is morning sunlight necessary and beneficial to the
mind, body, and spirit?

- Morning sunlight elevates your mood by boosting
  serotonin levels.
- It improves sleep by increasing nighttime melatonin
  production.
- It promotes bone growth through vitamin D activation.
- It strengthens the immune system and reduces infection
  rates.
- It lowers blood pressure and reduces the risk of stroke
  and heart disease.

- It may reduce melanoma and certain cancer risks.
- It promotes weight loss and lowers BMI.
- It enhances cognitive performance and improves quality of life.

Tip

Not everyone can get out into the sunshine within an hour of waking. If that is the case, sit near a window or use a light lamp. Be careful not to burn yourself or look directly at the sun.

Prayer

Triune God, You are like the sun, shining down Your love from above. Thank You for the healing effects of the sun and for the true healing that only You provide. Help us not to complain when the sun does not appear but rather thank You for each day it warms our faces. You give such great gifts!

Reflection

How can I switch up my morning routine to allow for morning sunlight? Am I able to get up fifteen to twenty minutes earlier to allow for the life-giving benefits of morning sunlight? Am I able to take a fifteen-minute morning break for a brisk walk outside?

....
....
....
....

Action Step

To help you incorporate sunlight into your routine, schedule a day within the next week to get at least ten minutes of morning sunlight. Increase from there, as it is beneficial to get morning sunlight each day.

O, Sunshine! The most precious
gold to be found on earth.

—Roman Payne

SLEEP

Do you not know that your bodies are
temples of the Holy Spirit, who is in you,
whom you have received from God? You are
not your own; you were bought at a price.
Therefore honor God with your bodies.
—1 Corinthians 6:19–20

HERE IS GOD reminding us yet again that we are to take care
of the body (temple) He has blessed us with.

For many years, when my kids kept me busy running most
days, I often plopped down in front of the TV around nine
o'clock in the evening with a glass of wine, settling in for "me
time." You know, that time when you can finally take a breath
and relax. Funny thing is, this routine wasn't doing anything
for me. Instead of heading to bed and getting the rest I needed
to feel and be my best the next day, I filled my body with a
known carcinogen and spent my evenings mindlessly numbing
out in front of the TV. Over time, this became a habit that was
difficult to break when I finally realized how detrimental it was
to my health. Now, most nights, I welcome my sleep routine
and relish the fact that I wake up with more energy and fewer
cravings and less irritability.

How do we honor our body? By giving it what it needs—sleep! Prioritizing sleep is an intentional choice that sets us up to make healthy decisions throughout the day. If there is one thing that influences our health, it's getting proper rest. According to Dr. Jason Fung, a single night of sleep deprivation can increase cortisol levels by more than 100 percent, and as mentioned earlier, chronic high cortisol has significant health consequences.

Unfortunately, many people continue to neglect the life-giving properties of a good night's sleep, while others find themselves struggling to achieve it. Quality sleep starts with good sleep hygiene and a consistent wind-down routine. See the Tip below for ways to promote restful sleep.

Why is sleep necessary and beneficial to the mind, body, and spirit?

- Sleep enhances mood and alleviates mental distress.
- It supports heart health by allowing the heart and blood pressure to rest.
- It regulates blood sugar and reduces the risk of type 2 diabetes.
- It improves cognitive function and memory consolidation.
- It strengthens the immune system and aids in tissue repair.
- It reduces stress and mitigates anxiety and depression.
- It enhances athletic performance through muscle recovery.
- It supports weight management by regulating appetite hormones.
- It reduces inflammation and prevents chronic health issues.
- It improves balance and reduces the risk of falls.
- It boosts energy levels and alertness.

- It enhances memory and executive functioning.
- It repairs tissues and promotes overall health.

Tip

Ways to promote restful sleep:

Morning sunlight: Exposure to natural light during the day helps regulate your sleep-wake cycle.

Avoid screens, intense exercise, alcohol, or eating two hours before bed (preferably three hours).

Designate your bedroom solely for sleep: Keep TVs and phones out of the bedroom.

Invest in a comfy bed and quality bedding: This will enhance your comfort and support relaxation.

Use blackout shades: Block out light to create a dark, sleep-friendly environment.

Turn off the router at night: Reduce electromagnetic exposure and distractions.

Establish a wind-down routine: Engage in calming activities at the same time each day, such as reading, journaling, prayer, taking a bath, or gentle stretching.

Prayer

Holy Spirit, forgive me for the times I have neglected to give my body what it truly needs: sleep. Without quality sleep, I will struggle to make good decisions that impact my relationships, health, and well-being. Help me to practice good sleep hygiene and implement and stick to an evening sleep routine that will set me up for success the next day.

Reflection

What changes can I make right away—perhaps cutting back or removing alcohol and refraining from eating at least two hours before bed—that will improve my sleep quality?

....

....

....

....

....

....

Action Step

Create a wind-down routine that you can put into place within the next week.

A good laugh and a long sleep are the
best cures in the doctor's book.
—Irish Proverb

MINDSET AND VISUALIZATION

> Finally, brothers and sisters, whatever is
> true, whatever is noble, whatever is right,
> whatever is pure, whatever is lovely, whatever
> is admirable—if anything is excellent or
> praiseworthy—think about such things.
> —Philippians 4:8

I'LL BE HONEST; I've never considered myself a "glass-half-full" kinda gal. You see, I have struggled with complaining, staying positive, and worrying. And while I do think I have come a long way, this is an area where I need daily reminders. Reminders that God has my back, and my worrying isn't going to change a thing. In fact, it's an absolute waste of time and a sin.

Visualization involves imagining the outcomes you want to achieve and the person you want to become. Spending time envisioning the woman I want to be and the life I want to live, while taking my thoughts captive when I start spiraling, has transformed me. This didn't happen overnight, and I'm reminded most days that I still have work to do!

Why is the proper mindset necessary and beneficial to the mind, body, and spirit?

- A proper mindset increases optimism and positive emotions by enhancing overall mood.
- It helps regulate negative emotions like anxiety and a feeling of being overwhelmed by improving emotional stability.
- It facilitates decision-making and problem solving by aiding cognitive processes.
- It aids in achieving goals by planning steps and anticipating obstacles effectively.
- It acts as a mental rehearsal for executing plans, ensuring more effective goal accomplishment.

Tip

Dream big and don't fear how others will respond. As Marianne Williamson says in *A Return to Love*, you are a child of God. Your playing small does not serve the world. There is nothing enlightened about shrinking so that other people won't feel insecure around you.

Prayer

Father, Son and Holy Spirit, please redirect my thoughts to things that are true, noble, right, pure, lovely, and praiseworthy. Too often, I dwell on my shortcomings and compare myself to others. Help me to see the woman Jesus created me to be, free from sin and perfect in the Father's eyes because of His death on the cross. When I visualize that woman, it gives me the courage to live my life according to Your will.

Reflection

Does my mindset need attention? Do I often find myself worrying, thinking negatively, or comparing myself to others?

....

....

....

....

....

....

....

....

....

....

Action Step

When you wake tomorrow morning, visualize the person you want to be and life you want to live. You can walk yourself through your day, implementing the practices in this devotional. Ask God to help you make it a reality.

Whether you think you can, or you
think you can't—you're right.
—Henry Ford

ACTS OF KINDNESS

Therefore, as God's chosen people, holy and
dearly loved, clothe yourselves with compassion,
kindness, humility, gentleness and patience.
—Colossians 3:12

I'LL NEVER FORGET the day the yellow sticky note was stuck to my car window. I had stopped to get some groceries, and when I returned to my car, I was greeted with this message: "In case no one has told you, you have an amazing smile." Random acts of kindness can make a huge difference in the receiver's and the giver's life. While I loved this day brightener, I also love to do little things for others.

Why are acts of kindness necessary and beneficial to the mind, body, and spirit?

- Acts of kindness increase happiness and contentment by boosting personal joy.
- They enhance gratitude by fostering a sense of interconnectedness and appreciation.
- They deepen empathy and compassion by strengthening community and reducing feelings of isolation.

- They reduce stress and improve health by lowering negative emotions and strengthening the immune system.
- They release positive neurochemicals by reducing pain and enhancing social bonds through dopamine, serotonin, and oxytocin.
- They cultivate positivity by generating positive feelings in both givers and receivers.
- They encourage reciprocal acts of kindness by creating a ripple effect of positive actions.
- They humanize and elevate spiritual well-being by providing emotional support and fostering a habit of giving.

Tip

An act of kindness can be any simple act that will make someone feel special. A simple smile or greeting when you meet someone. A card or letter in the mail just because you were thinking of them. A meal for a sick or busy friend.

Of special note, many struggle with ways to help the homeless. One way I have helped is to hand out mini Bibles or a devotional with a bottle of water. They may toss it in the garbage, or they might be touched by someone who loves God also showing love to them.

Prayer

Dear Jesus, thanks for the ultimate act of kindness when You died on the cross for our sins. May we never forget Your sacrifice and show our appreciation by loving others through acts of kindness. The cool thing is that we benefit as well. Thanks for this wonderful blessing.

Reflection

What is one act of kindness I can do this week? Is this something I can see myself making a daily, weekly, or even monthly practice?

....
....
....
....
....
....
....
....
....
....
....

Action Step

Smile at a stranger today. It benefits you both!

Random acts of kindness cost
nothing but mean everything.
—Unknown

GRATITUDE

Give thanks in all circumstances; for this
is God's will for you in Christ Jesus.
—1 Thessalonians 5:18

THE BOOK ONE *Thousand Gifts* by Ann Voskamp clearly demonstrates how being grateful can change your life. It also brought to my attention how I had failed miserably at being grateful. How many times did I forget to go back to God and thank Him for an answered prayer? How many prayers started with more and more requests versus praising Him for who He was and what He had already done in my blessed life? I tear up when I listen to Seph Schlueter's song "Counting My Blessings." When we thank God for what He has done, we switch the focus from us to Him. The most awesome gift giver of all.

Why is gratitude necessary and beneficial to the mind, body, and spirit?

- Gratitude enhances your overall mood and increases optimism by fostering positive feelings and reducing stress.
- It improves sleep by reducing negative emotions and promoting a sense of well-being.
- It boosts immunity and lowers disease risk by triggering positive physiological responses and enhancing overall health.

- It decreases depression and anxiety by practicing daily gratitude and shifting focus away from discomfort.
- It reduces difficulties with chronic pain by improving overall well-being and managing discomfort.
- It strengthens social connections and improves relationships by releasing oxytocin and fostering mutual positivity.
- It increases resilience and encourages the development of patience, humility, and wisdom.
- It lowers levels of cellular inflammation and reduces fatigue by promoting better physical health.
- It enhances job satisfaction and employee effectiveness by improving relationships and prosocial behaviors in the workplace.
- It improves cognitive functions such as decision-making and problem solving by enhancing emotional stability and focus.

Tip

Make a conscious effort and ask God to help you recognize when you are complaining. When you catch yourself, ask for forgiveness and find something to be thankful for instead.

Prayer

Dear Lord, first and foremost, I should be thanking and praising You for what You have done regardless of the health benefits gratitude provides me. But in true God fashion, You bless us when we bless You. Help me to always be grateful, in the good times and in the bad. Help me to remember that Your ways are higher than mine and that You work out everything for good. Thank You for all the answered prayers and blessings. You amaze me with Your generosity!

Reflection

Do I lean more toward complaining rather than giving thanks? What are you most grateful for?

....
....
....
....
....
....
....
....
....
....

Action Step

Start a gratitude jar. Place a small slip of paper in a mason jar each week listing something you are grateful for. On January 1, take them out and read them and praise God for His generosity.

Gratitude is a powerful catalyst for happiness. It's
the spark that lights a fire of joy in your soul.
—Robert Emmons

PRAYER

Do not be anxious about anything, but in every
situation, by prayer and petition, with thanksgiving,
present your requests to God. And the peace of
God, which transcends all understanding, will
guard your hearts and your minds in Christ Jesus.
—Philippians 4:6–7

PRAYER HAS ALWAYS been an important part of my life,
whether I was seeking help for a lost bracelet (which miraculously
turned up on my cousin's driveway), praying for my volleyball
serve to clear the net, or asking for guidance during exams
and in relationships. Looking back at my high school journal, I
often cringe at some entries, but I smile at the prayers scribbled
in the margins. Knowing I've laid my concerns at the feet of the
one who made the heavens and the earth brings so much peace.

Why is prayer necessary and beneficial to the mind, body,
and spirit?

- Prayer enhances overall well-being by fostering a deeper
  sense of purpose and meaning beyond daily life.
- It provides emotional support by connecting individuals
  with like-minded communities, reducing loneliness
  and boosting resilience.

- It improves mood by promoting positive emotions, better emotional processing, and increased feelings of forgiveness and purpose.
- It helps you to cope with challenges by offering a spiritual framework for managing difficult situations, such as loss and grief.
- It cultivates gratitude through prayer, decreasing negative emotions and contributing to better overall health.
- It encourages mindfulness by focusing on present-moment awareness, reducing stress, and fostering a sense of peace.
- It supports physical healing and heart health, with evidence showing its positive impact on cardiovascular health and recovery from illness.
- It induces relaxation by lowering stress levels, heart rate, and blood pressure, and alleviates symptoms of various conditions.

Tip

God tells us in His word that the Lord's Prayer is a perfect place to start when it comes to prayer. Keep in mind that as much as God loves to hear our requests, He also appreciates gratitude and thankfulness.

Prayer

Heavenly Father, thank You so much for the privilege to come to You in prayer. I can't believe that I have access to the one and only true God. I love that I can come to You at any time, and You will hear me. It brings comfort, joy, and peace.

Reflection

Do I only go to God in time of need, or am I communicating with Him multiple times a day as I would with anyone here on earth who is important to me?

....

....

....

....

....

....

....

....

....

....

Action Step

Experiment with starting each prayer with praise. When I go to God, I like to acknowledge a quality of His and praise Him for it (I learned this from author Lisa Whelchel). Then I thank Him for His many blessings and bring Him my requests.

Is prayer your steering wheel or your spare tire?
—Corrie Ten Boom

JOURNALING
(PRAYER AND PERSONAL)

I will remember the deeds of the Lord;
yes, I will remember your miracles of long
ago. I will consider all your works and
meditate on all your mighty deeds.
—Psalm 77:11–12

JOURNALING ISN'T SOMETHING I've mastered. I have multiple journals, but many only have a few pages filled. Although I start with the best intentions, I often struggle to make it a priority. Nonetheless, I cherish revisiting those pages, where I discover answered prayers, cherished memories, and messages from God.

One of my sweetest childhood memories is finding my grandma's journals, which clearly reflected her deep love for and trust in God. I hope to improve my journaling practice, and I genuinely hope that my kids and grandkids will enjoy my journals as much as I cherished my grandmother's.

Why is journaling necessary and beneficial to the mind, body, and spirit?

- Journaling reduces stress and anxiety by allowing you to process and express your feelings through writing.

- It enhances creativity by stimulating imagination and capturing ideas for future projects.
- It improves memory by reflecting on past experiences, aiding in retention and serving as a reminder of meaningful events.
- It boosts self-awareness by increasing understanding of your thoughts and emotions, leading to personal growth.
- It promotes good mental health by helping manage symptoms of depression and other conditions through coping and processing feelings.
- It increases motivation by tracking goals and progress, helping to maintain focus and drive.
- It provides a sense of accomplishment as completing entries offers satisfaction and a record of personal growth over time.
- It strengthens relationships by enhancing understanding and communication and fostering gratitude and appreciation.
- It increases productivity by helping prioritize tasks and plans, leading to better organization.
- It creates a legacy by leaving a lasting record for future generations, offering insights into your life and personality.

Tip ───────────────────────────────────

Pick out a pretty journal and fancy pen. Keep them out in the open or near a chair you frequent so you are more likely to use them. While some people use their phones to take notes or to journal, I believe the actual act of writing (regardless of if you can read the writing, which is sometimes the case for me) makes it even more special and beneficial.

I recently began using a pocket-sized prayer journal to track my prayer requests. It fits perfectly in my purse! In the past, I would often promise to pray for others but forget because I didn't jot it down. This new approach has been a game changer for me.

Prayer

Holy God, even though I may not be the best at journaling, thanks for the times You gently nudge me to take the time to write down my thoughts, feelings, prayers, and blessings. I love looking back at my journals and seeing all the ways You have blessed me and my family and friends. You are absolutely amazing!

Reflection

Is journaling something I currently enjoy? When would be a good time to engage in this practice?

....
....
....
....
....
....
....
....
....
....

Action Step

Pick up or order a pretty journal and fancy pen and start journaling.

Preserve your memories, keep them well,
what you forget you can never retell.
—Louisa May Alcott

PLAY (DANCING OR OTHER HOBBIES)

A time to weep, and a time to laugh; a
time to mourn, and a time to dance.
—Ecclesiastes 3:4

GROWING UP ON a farm, and having a Scandinavian and German heritage, I often overlooked play in favor of hard work. My work ethic was frequently praised, which led me to believe that "playing" wasn't something to be prioritized or valued. During a visit to a monastery in Spain, I even contemplated getting a tattoo that read "work and pray" in Latin, symbolizing my deeply ingrained belief in hard work over play. But over time, I realized that all work and no play makes Patty a dysregulated girl.

While I've always loved dancing (which goes hand in hand with my love for music), I recently discovered that dancing isn't just good for physical health—it also helps regulate the nervous system. I used to think that the only way to regulate my nervous system was through stillness—by being quiet, reflecting, and meditating. But I learned that this only works if you're in a sympathetic state. When you're in a freeze or shut-down state, you need the exact opposite. So, now when I'm feeling overwhelmed or unmotivated, I turn up my favorite songs and allow the music to move me however my body needs to in that moment. Why is play necessary and beneficial to the mind, body, and spirit?

- Play releases endorphins, which promote a sense of well-being, provide temporary pain relief, and enhance emotional healing by replacing negative behaviors with positive interactions.
- It enhances brain function and memory while helping to prevent stress and depression. It encourages a playful mindset that makes learning more efficient and enjoyable.
- It fosters imagination, problem-solving skills, and creativity, making learning new tasks more enjoyable and effective, and enhances work productivity by boosting creativity, teamwork, and job satisfaction while reducing stress and burnout.
- It improves empathy, trust, intimacy, and social skills, helping to develop new friendships and business relationships and promoting social bonding.
- It increases energy levels, making you feel more youthful, and supports resilience against illness. Staying playful keeps you feeling vibrant and counteracts the effects of aging.

Tip

Make a playlist on Spotify of your favorite upbeat songs (I include secular and praise songs). The next time you are feeling overwhelmed or even stuck, get up, crank the songs from your playlist, and dance. You'll be amazed at how it lifts your mood and energizes your body. If dancing isn't your thing, make time to participate in something you love doing.

Prayer

Creator God, thank You for the gift of play, whether that be dance, singing, playing an instrument, or just a favorite hobby. You say in Your word that there is a time for everything. Remind me that play isn't just OK; I was made to play and will benefit from it in so many ways.

Reflection

Do I currently take time to "play"? What are some play activities that I would enjoy?

....

....

....

....

....

....

....

....

....

....

....

....

....

Action Step

Schedule a play date for this coming week or experiment with using dance as a stress reliever.

We don't stop playing because we grow old;
we grow old because we stop playing.
—George Bernard Shaw

NATURE AND GROUNDING

The heavens declare the glory of God; the
skies proclaim the work of his hands.
—Psalm 19:1

WHILE SOME MIGHT say that nature could be included in movement and play, I think it deserves its own mention. Nature is my happy place. It is where I feel closest to God. Once when I was away at college, I drove three hours, lay in the grass at our farm for an hour and turned around and headed back. I can't emphasize enough the calm and joy the trees, birds, hills, creeks, and valleys bring to my mind, body, and soul.

Why is spending time in nature necessary and beneficial to the mind, body, and spirit?

- Time in nature lowers stress levels by calming the sympathetic nervous system, which reduces blood pressure, heart rate, and blood sugar and enhances relaxation by clearing the mind for deeper thinking.
- It improves mood by alleviating feelings of anxiety, depression, and irritability, and promotes emotional well-being by helping us manage emotions like loneliness and improving overall emotional health.

- It boosts cognitive function by enhancing memory, attention span, creativity, and sleep quality while also supporting mental health conditions such as PTSD, ADHD, and anxiety disorders.
- It increases resiliency and promotes self-care, helping us to manage the demands of daily life.

Tip

If you can't easily access nature, try grounding. Step outside, kick off your shoes, and dig your toes into the earth. No grass in sight? Surround yourself with nature-inspired art, indoor plants, or natural objects like rocks and sticks.

Prayer

Triune God, thank You for this beautiful earth You created. It screams of Your glory and brings health benefits as well. Nature is such a gift. Help me to always respect and take care of this gift.

Reflection

Am I spending time in nature and respecting the earth God created?

....
....
....
....

Action Step

Slip off those shoes and head out for a grounding session. Even better, schedule a hike with or without a friend and admire the gorgeous world we live in.

I love to think of nature as an unlimited broadcasting station through which God speaks to us every hour, if we only will tune in.
—George Washington Carver

BREATHWORK

The Spirit of God has made me; the
breath of the Almighty gives me life.
—Job 33:4

THIS VERSE SPEAKS of breath giving life, and that it truly
does. Breathwork has helped me when things get challenging. I
use it when I start to feel the panic coming on and when I wake
in the middle of the night and my mind starts racing. It helps
me to stay present and not worry about mistakes in the past or
risks in the future.

A trick I learned from the creator of the Success Solution
and my mentor Debra Joy is to focus more on the exhale.
This activates the parasympathetic nervous system, which
decreases heart rate, lowers blood pressure, promotes
relaxation, and helps the body calm down and recover from
stress.

Why is breathwork necessary and beneficial to the mind,
body, and spirit?

- Breathwork helps manage stress and anxiety
  by completing the stress cycle and grounding
  individuals in the present, countering the fight-or-
  flight response.

- It enhances oxygen intake, boosting energy levels and strengthening the immune system, thus mitigating the effects of stress on health.
- It aids in reducing blood pressure and improving circulation by activating the parasympathetic nervous system and relaxing blood vessels.
- It can alleviate pain and discomfort by promoting relaxation and providing distraction, positively influencing mood and stress levels.
- It improves lung capacity and respiratory function, benefiting those with chronic conditions and enhancing overall lung health.
- It can elevate mood, boost self-confidence, and enhance self-perception by reducing stress and fostering a sense of inner peace.
- It helps expel toxins from the body, improves oxygenation, and supports the lymphatic system, contributing to overall detoxification.
- It can regulate energy levels and aid in falling asleep, serving as a natural remedy for insomnia and sleep disturbances.
- It can support the management of depression by altering mood and enhancing emotional well-being.
- It supports muscle tone improvement by alkalizing the blood and enhancing muscle contractions, which benefits physical performance.
- It can be a therapeutic tool for dealing with trauma and PTSD, helping to manage symptoms and foster emotional healing.
- It aids in digestive health by increasing blood flow to the digestive tract, reducing stress, and supporting better digestive function.

- It can be beneficial in addiction recovery by providing calm and focus, assisting in managing cravings, and enhancing self-awareness.
- It enhances concentration and attention span by calming the mind and affecting the brain's chemical messengers related to focus.
- It can boost creativity and problem-solving abilities by relaxing the mind and allowing new ideas to flow.

Tip

There are many ways to practice breathwork. I find it best to start slow. Box breathing is a great place to start. When confronted with a stressful situation, breathe in through the nose for a count of four and hold your breath for a count of four. Then breathe out for a count of four and hold your breath for a count of four. Complete four rounds and see how you feel.

Prayer

Dearest Jesus, breath is life. Help me to prioritize slowing down enough to really breathe. Many days I am rushing from sunrise to sunset without taking time to receive the health benefits proper breathing provides. This is a simple practice that is free and takes little time. When I care for myself, I can serve You better.

Reflection ————————————————

Sit quietly and observe your breathing. Are you taking short, shallow breaths, or are you inhaling deeply, supplying your body with the oxygen it needs to function effectively.

....

....

....

....

....

....

....

....

....

....

Action Step ————————————————

Look up the four/seven/eight breathwork technique and utilize it the next time you have trouble falling asleep or wake in the middle of the night.

When you own your breath, nobody
can steal your peace.
—Author unknown

STAYING PRESENT

Therefore do not worry about tomorrow,
for tomorrow will worry about itself. Each
day has enough trouble of its own.
—Matthew 6:34

AS A CARD-CARRYING member of the "Control Patrol," I have had to work hard to embrace staying present. I mentioned earlier that worry has often overshadowed joy in my life. I thought that if everything was planned and organized, I would be prepared and in control. I spent countless hours on to-do lists, planning, and looking to the future instead of enjoying and being thankful for what God had given me at that moment.

Living in the present helps us avoid focusing on past regrets or future worries, which can alleviate stress and feelings of being overwhelmed.

Why is staying present necessary and beneficial to the mind, body, and spirit?

- Staying focused on the present helps alleviate stress and anxiety, reducing mood swings and contributing to overall mental well-being.
- It enhances self-awareness, allowing for a better understanding of your emotions and surroundings.

- It improves your ability to listen and connect with others, fostering more meaningful relationships.
- It enhances work performance by minimizing distractions and reducing mistakes.
- It allows you to fully appreciate and enjoy everyday experiences, leading to increased happiness.
- It aids in absorbing information more effectively and developing skills without being hindered by past failures or future fears.

Tip

When we live in the present moment, it is impossible to worry about the past or future. I use a little trick my mentor Debra Joy taught me, called FAB. I refer to this practice as SAP—as I added prayer.

First, sit in a chair. Then scan (S) your body; feel your feet on the floor, your bottom in the chair, and your breath. Focus on your airway (A); slowly breathe in through your nose to a count of four, then exhale (focusing here) to a count of eight. You can also add in prayer (P) when you switch from inhale to exhale. Perhaps repeat a mantra like "You are awesome, God," "Help me to stay present," or "Thank you, Jesus." I always feel calmer when I pray, so I added that to Debra's original FAB.

Prayer

Heavenly Father, forgive me for trying to control my life with obsessive planning and not trusting what You have in store for me. Help me to live in the present and enjoy all the wonderful blessings You provide each and every day.

Reflection ——————————————

Am I also a card-carrying member of the Control Patrol? Am I guilty of dwelling in the past or dreaming of the future instead of living in the present moment?

....

....

....

....

....

....

....

....

....

....

Action Step ——————————————

To take it a step further than just a breathwork practice, the next time you start to feel stressed or overwhelmed, use the SAP technique to bring you into the present and notice as you begin to feel calmer and less stressed.

There are only two days in the year that nothing
can be done. One is called yesterday, and the
other is called tomorrow, so today is the right
day to love, believe, do, and mostly live.
—Dalai Lama

YOGA (SACRED STRETCH)

> But those who hope in the LORD will renew
> their strength. They will soar on wings
> like eagles; they will run and not grow
> weary, they will walk and not be faint.
> —Isaiah 40:31

I REMEMBER THE first time my friend Johanna invited me to yoga. I thought, *I am going to* hate *it. I can't be bothered with just lying around and stretching.* I had no idea what yoga was really about. In time I have come to *love* yoga. I enjoy slowing down and living in the present. While sometimes I have a hard time keeping my mind from wandering, there is no judgment.

I will say that I practice yoga a bit differently than what is intended (I call this sacred stretch). I'm not at one with the universe, but rather at one with my Father in heaven. I often pray during savasana and give thanks for the opportunity to move my body and strengthen my mind.

Why is yoga, or what I like to call sacred stretch, necessary and beneficial to the mind, body, and spirit?

- Yoga enhances muscular strength, balance, and flexibility through controlled movements and deep breathing exercises.

- It can alleviate lower back pain and improve mobility, making it an effective approach for managing chronic back discomfort.
- It helps reduce discomfort and improve mobility in individuals with arthritis.
- It may lower stress and inflammation, supporting heart health and addressing risk factors like high blood pressure and excess weight.
- It can help prepare your body for restful sleep and improve overall sleep quality.
- It boosts both physical and mental energy, enhances alertness, and improves mood.
- It supports effective stress management and mental well-being by promoting mindfulness and relaxation.
- It can reduce feelings of loneliness and foster a supportive environment, enhancing social connections and group healing.
- It has benefits across various health areas, reinforcing its role in overall self-care and well-being.

Tip

I have cheap yoga mats in my bedroom, office, and on my porch so I can drop down anytime of the day!

My very favorite yoga pose is Child's Pose. You simply get down on the floor on all fours, sink your bottom back and stretch your hands out in front of you. It is so calming, and it is a great stretch as well. I intend to start each day in this pose, offering a prayer of gratitude for the restorative sleep I received and for the strength and protection I need for the day ahead.

Prayer

Father God, while I don't adhere to all the teachings of traditional yoga, I do enjoy the benefits of the practice. I welcome the time to slow down and enjoy the present moment and the strength and beauty of the body You have blessed me with, flaws and all. I also find that it is a great time to check in with You and to praise and thank You for the many gifts You have so graciously given.

Reflection

If yoga isn't part of your routine yet, do you feel more inclined to try it after learning about its many benefits for the mind, body, and spirit?

....

....

....

....

....

Action Step

Check out "Yoga by Adrienne" on YouTube. She is great for beginners and advanced yogis as well. I also encourage you to support your local Yoga studio.

> Yoga is not about touching your toes, it's
> about what you learn on the way down.
> —Sadhguru

CONTENTMENT

But godliness with contentment is great
gain. For we brought nothing into the world,
and we can take nothing out of it.
—1 Timothy 6:6–7

WHILE SOME MAY view contentment solely in terms of material possessions, I also look at it as it relates to "self-acceptance." Are you content when you are not working or producing? Can you sit with yourself without scrolling on your phone or listening to a podcast or music? Are you accepting of your body?

I have struggled with understanding that my worth comes from being a child of God, which has made contentment a challenge for me. I now stand firm, knowing I am not defined by my job title, how much I got done on my to-do list, or the size of my waist.

We are also called to be content with material possessions. Remember God's words in Job 1:21: "The LORD gave and the LORD has taken away; may the name of the LORD be praised."

Why is contentment necessary and beneficial to the mind, body, and spirit?

- Contentment helps lower stress levels, improving overall health and preventing stress-related conditions. Reduced stress and improved mood are linked to lower blood pressure and a decreased risk of heart disease.
- It contributes to a stronger immune system, reducing susceptibility to illnesses.
- It can lead to better sleep by reducing anxiety and worry that disrupt rest.
- It alleviates symptoms of depression and anxiety, contributing to better mental health.
- It is associated with a longer life due to improved overall health and reduced risk of chronic diseases.
- It fosters emotional resilience, leading to a more balanced and stable mental state.
- It can lead to healthier, more supportive relationships, benefiting overall well-being.

Tip

This has proven to be one of the most difficult practices for me. It has taken some time to be able to find contentment through slowing down and enjoying everyday activities and experiences, whether it's enjoying a cup of coffee (without scrolling on my phone), taking a walk (without headphones), or spending time with loved ones. Be kind and patient with yourself and have realistic expectations. None of this happens overnight. As I say to all my clients: Progress over perfection!

Prayer

Giver of all gifts, forgive me for the times where I have not been content. Help me to see that the simpler life is, the more time there is to focus on You and the wonderful family and friends You have blessed me with. I don't need to work more to get more, but rather be content with what I already have (both with myself and with my possessions), which is way more than I will ever need.

Reflection

Do I slow down enough to enjoy the little things in life? Does working more to buy more stuff (or to earn my worth) really merit what I'm missing out on in the process—especially time with You?

....

....

....

....

....

....

....

Action Step

The next time you head out on a walk, leave your headphones at home. Make an effort to just take everything in and be with yourself.

The secret of happiness, you see, is
not found in seeking more, but in
developing the capacity to enjoy less.
—Socrates

BOUNDARIES

Moses' father-in-law replied, 'What you are doing
is not good. You and these people who come to
you will only wear yourselves out. The work is
too heavy for you; you cannot handle it alone.'
—Exodus 18:17–18

BOUNDARIES HELP KEEP things simpler and calmer in life. For years I didn't know how to say no, and I was overwhelmed and physically and emotionally exhausted. I was a grade A people pleaser and didn't want to disappoint. However, after I realized how detrimental having no boundaries is to health, I decided it was time to reevaluate where I was actually needed. I got comfortable saying what author Chalene Johnson recommends: "I'm not sure that is going to work; let me check my calendar and get back to you." I slowly but surely made a conscious effort to not overfill my days and relished in the peace quiet days resting gave to my body and soul.

Throughout His ministry, Jesus frequently faced requests for His time, attention, and resources. However, He demonstrated remarkable discernment by saying no when necessary. This ability to set boundaries was not rooted in selfishness but in a profound understanding of His purpose and mission. By modeling this behavior, Jesus teaches us that boundaries are not merely barriers; they are essential components of living a focused and intentional life. When we learn to say no, we create space for what truly matters—our relationship with God, our health and personal growth, and our ability to serve others wholeheartedly. In a world that often demands our time and energy, we can look to Jesus as our guide, recognizing that saying no is sometimes the most loving thing we can do—for ourselves and those we serve.

Why is boundary setting necessary and beneficial to the mind, body, and spirit?

- Establishing clear boundaries helps manage personal and professional responsibilities, leading to reduced stress and increased satisfaction in life.
- They enhance overall contentment by clearly defining roles and responsibilities in various relationships.
- They prevent anxiety by avoiding the absorption of others' emotions, behaviors, and thoughts.
- They clarify where your responsibilities end and others' begin, promoting healthier and more balanced interactions.
- They reinforce your sense of self-worth, independent of external validation or performance.
- They improve relationships by fostering mutual respect and reducing feelings of mistreatment or exploitation.
- They support personal growth and alignment with your values and goals.
- They strengthen your ability to protect your well-being and avoid overcommitment.
- They effectively improve interpersonal dynamics and reduce misunderstandings.
- They build resilience over time, reduce the pressure to please others, and enhance self-esteem and overall well-being.

Tip

I recommend a book like *Boundaries* by Henry Cloud and John Townsend to get you started on your journey. This can seem daunting at first, but actually becomes much easier. I was blown away by the difference in my life when I started to say no. Did I disappoint some? Yes. But I also felt less stressed, and as a result, I ultimately had more to give to others because I was happier and healthier.

Prayer

Oh God, thank You so much for helping me to see that I don't need to say yes to everyone and everything and that slowing down and caring for myself will benefit those I love and in the long run is the best for everyone. While this can be challenging and take time for others to understand and respect, help me stand firm in my convictions and convey my boundaries to others in a respectful and gentle way. You are the only one I aim to impress, and Your opinion is ultimately the only one that matters.

Reflection:

Do I have proper boundaries in place, or am I consistently putting others' needs before my own? What small step can I take today to establish better boundaries?

....

....

....

....

Action Step

The next time someone asks you to do something for them, practice "Let me check my calendar and get back to you."

Boundaries are not about separation, but about defining our values, our priorities, and our calling.

—Ruth Haley Barton

LAUGHTER

A cheerful heart is good medicine, but
a crushed spirit dries up the bones.
—Proverbs 17:22

LAST FALL I organized a trip with a bunch of my high school friends to see comedian Leanne Morgan. Not only did I benefit from the joy and healing aspect of community, but we also laughed so hard that our stomachs hurt. Had I not slowed down and said no to several other "obligations," I would have missed out on that healing weekend with lifelong friends.

While my frown lines certainly outnumber my laugh lines, I'm bound and determined to make smiling and laughter a bigger part of my day-to-day life.

Why is laughter necessary and beneficial to the mind, body, and spirit?

- Laughing stimulates multiple organs by increasing oxygen intake and enhancing the function of your heart, lungs, and muscles, while boosting endorphin release.
- It activates and then calms your stress response, leading to a temporary rise and subsequent decrease

in heart rate and blood pressure, resulting in a relaxed feeling.

- It helps reduce tension by improving circulation and relaxing muscles, which alleviates some physical symptoms of stress.
- It can strengthen your immune system by counteracting stress-induced chemical reactions and releasing neuropeptides that combat stress and illness.
- It can help relieve pain by promoting the production of the body's natural painkillers.
- It increases personal satisfaction by making it easier to handle difficult situations and enhancing social connections.
- It improves mood and can alleviate symptoms of depression and anxiety, contributing to a greater sense of happiness and higher self-esteem.

Tip

Just like laughter, smiling is beneficial to your health. Forcing a smile can trick your brain into feeling happier, even if you're not initially in a good mood. This is due to the feedback loop between facial expressions and emotions. So, even if you don't feel like it, try forcing yourself to smile.

Prayer

Dear Lord, thank You so much for the gift of laughter. Forgive me for when I have taken things too seriously which has resulted in deep frown lines and very few laugh lines. Help me bring laughter to others and make (take) time to enjoy fun activities with friends and family.

Reflection

Do you think you could benefit from more laughter or turning your frown upside down?

....

....

....

....

....

....

....

....

....

Action Step

Experiment with smiling when you least feel like smiling. Did you notice any difference? Pull up a YouTube video of Leanne Morgan or Nate Bargatze for a good laugh.

Laughter is the most beautiful and beneficial
therapy God ever granted humanity.
—Deepak Chopra

COMMUNITY

Therefore encourage one another and build
each other up, just as in fact you are doing.
—1 Thessalonians 5:11

I HAVE BEEN greatly blessed by Christian family and friends my entire life. At every stage of life, I could reach out for Christian advice. When we moved away from friends in Minnesota, I was blessed to find next-door neighbors and other friends who sent their children to the same Christian school system. These new friendships quickly became my family here in Wisconsin.

Though God made us for community, as an introvert, I sometimes find this challenging. However, God has worked on my heart, and I now realize how vital community is for my spiritual, physical, and emotional health.

Why is community necessary and beneficial to the mind, body, and spirit?

- Being part of a community fosters a sense of belonging, which is essential for psychological well-being and helps individuals feel connected to something greater than themselves.

- It offers emotional assistance, practical help, and advice, reducing feelings of isolation and providing comfort during difficult times.
- It helps develop a sense of identity by sharing values, beliefs, and cultural history, reinforcing one's place in the world.
- It can lower stress levels and feelings of isolation, contributing to better physical health, such as reduced blood pressure and cholesterol, and promoting a healthy lifestyle.
- It can enhance social support and alleviate feelings of loneliness, fostering overall mental health and well-being.

Tip

If you are already attending a church, join a small group Bible study or volunteer to get to know others better. Online Christian communities can be particularly helpful for introverts or those unable to attend in-person gatherings.

Prayer

Father, Son, and Holy Spirit, what incredible blessings friendship and community bring. I'm especially thankful for the Christian friends You have brought into every stage of my life. Help me to be a good friend and witness my faith in whatever community I am a part of.

Reflection

Am I more inclined to stay to myself, or do I actively engage in community with others? Now that I understand the health benefits of community, how can I become more involved in my church, neighborhood, or other organizations?

....

....

....

....

....

....

....

Action Step

If you aren't actively part of a church community, organization or friend group, research something that sounds interesting to you. Is there a Bible study coming up at church? Is there a neighborhood watch group or an organization where you could volunteer? Commit to attending at least one meeting to see if it's a good fit.

Most of the issues you face in life can be solved
with one of these three things: a walk outside, a
good night's sleep and a conversation with a friend.
—Mel Robbins

DIGITAL DETOX

Do not conform to the pattern of this world, but
be transformed by the renewing of your mind.
Then you will be able to test and approve what
God's will is—his good, pleasing and perfect will.
—Romans 12:2

I COULD PROBABLY write an entire book on this subject alone. Most people are aware of the negative effects technology is having on our world. While there are obviously benefits of technology, it comes down to balance.

I experienced this firsthand last year when I took a trip up to the Boundary Waters with extended family. While the scenery is breathtaking, and the company was great, the very best thing about the trip was that I had no access to my phone or computer. Days included meals around the fire, hikes, canoeing, fishing, hanging in the hammock, and just *being*! I felt like a different person after I returned, and I vowed to start limiting my technology use. While I still have a lot of room for improvement, this is something I need to focus on if I want to experience the numerous health benefits of a digital detox.

Why is a digital detox necessary and beneficial to the mind, body, and spirit?

- A digital detox can reduce stress levels and improve overall contentment by allowing you to focus on the present moment and engage more fully with your surroundings.
- It can enhance productivity by minimizing distractions and allowing more time to complete essential tasks and responsibilities.
- It can boost self-esteem by reducing the negative effects of constant social media comparisons, leading to a more positive self-image.
- It can alleviate physical discomforts such as eye strain, headaches, and musculoskeletal issues caused by prolonged screen use.
- It can improve sleep quality by reducing exposure to screens before bedtime, which helps regulate sleep cycles and promotes better rest.

Tip

My number one tip is to turn off any notifications. Every time you get a notification on your computer, phone, or watch, you are stimulating your nervous system. We were not made to get interrupted by these notifications day in and day out.

I would also advise powering your phone off or putting it on airplane mode during the workday. You can schedule a couple times to check messages to be sure nothing is an emergency. This will benefit your health and help you to be much more productive during the day.

Prayer

Dear God, while I understand that technology has its benefits, I pray for the strength to use it wisely and not allow it to consume my life. Remind me to take scheduled breaks away from my phone and especially social media. Help me to not fall into the comparison trap that social media promotes and to be content with the life and body You have blessed me with.

Reflection

Do I spend too much time on my phone? What could I be doing instead that would bring me closer to my family, friends, and God?

....
....
....
....
....
....
....
....
....
....
....
....
....

Action Step

Track how much time you spend on your phone for a few days. Most phones have a setting where you can monitor your screen time. Are you OK with that number? How are you going to change it?

Disconnecting from the digital world
can help us reconnect with the world
around us and with ourselves.
—Jaron Lanier

CHRISTIAN MEDITATION

Come near to God and He will come near to you.
—James 4:8

I'VE HAD A Christian meditation (quiet time) practice where I read different devotionals and converse with God for many, many years. However, I didn't make it a priority. It was usually the first thing to go when things got busy. I often thought to myself, *I just don't have time today.* I started questioning that idea when I consistently "found" more time when I decided to sit down and do quiet time (even if only for a few minutes) instead of skipping it. The days I would prioritize it, even when it was a full day, would lead to God blessing me with more time in my day. It was wild!

How can we expect to draw nearer to God if we don't make learning about Him and spending time with Him a priority? If you wanted to grow closer to someone, wouldn't spending time with them be essential? The same is true for God.

Even the busiest person can prioritize a few minutes each day to spend with God. While I like to do it first thing in the morning, find where it works for you. Perhaps at lunch or before bed. Hopefully you will soon be increasing the time spent in Christian meditation as you experience firsthand the benefits of this practice.

Why is Christian meditation necessary and beneficial to the mind, body, and spirit?

- Engaging in Christian meditation and mindfulness can alleviate stress and anxiety by fostering a focus on the present moment and reducing future worries and past regrets, which enhances overall tranquility.
- It improves concentration and productivity by training the mind to remain present, leading to increased mental clarity and better performance in daily tasks and personal development.
- It enhances emotional well-being by promoting gratitude, contentment, and self-compassion, resulting in improved self-esteem and more fulfilling relationships.
- It can strengthen the immune system and reduce inflammation, positively impacting physical health and aiding in the prevention of chronic illnesses.
- It can deepen your spiritual connection by providing time for reflection and prayer, helping you understand God's will and experience His presence more profoundly.
- It cultivates a spirit of gratitude and contentment, increasing your overall joy and satisfaction in life.
- It enhances discernment and wisdom, enabling you to make informed decisions and navigate life's challenges with greater clarity.
- It fosters compassion and forgiveness by encouraging you to view others through God's eyes, improving relationships through extended grace and understanding.

Tip

A great place to start is with a devotional such as *Jesus Calling* by Sarah Young or any devotional that resonates with you. From there you can add more time and additional practices like the Bible App or even just reading a few verses each day in the Bible. Listening to worship songs can add a whole new element to your quiet time. Don't forget to start off by praising God for who He is and thanking Him for all that He has done for you.

Consider creating a designated space for your quiet time where your devotions, Bible, and materials are easily accessible and visible. Make it part of your morning routine, and if you don't have a routine, this is a great place to start.

Prayer

Most amazing, perfect, and powerful God, first off thanks so much for being so huge that I don't have to worry about a thing. I know that You direct my path and work out everything for my good. Please help me to prioritize my quiet time with You each and every day. What could possibly take precedence over spending time with the one and only true God?

Reflection

Am I making my relationship with God a priority by spending time in His Word and in His presence? What obstacles are preventing me from doing so, and how can I address them?

....

....

....

....

....

....

Action Step

This week, set aside at least five minutes each day for Christian meditation. Choose a time that works best for you and schedule it in your calendar, setting an alarm to remind you.

God's voice is often heard in the quietness of
our hearts, not in the noise of the world.
—Anonymous

NOURISHMENT

So whether you eat or drink or whatever
you do, do it all for the glory of God.
—1 Corinthians 10:31

THIS LAST PRACTICE is separated into three sections. I recommend taking one a day, but you can tackle them all at once if you choose to do so.

Clean Food

While my diet today is primarily full of whole, quality foods including but not limited to grass-fed beef; pasture-raised eggs, pork, and chicken; wild-caught fish; and organic veggies, roots, and fruits, that was not always the case. Before I became a nutritional therapy practitioner, I was interested in food, but for the wrong reason. I was looking for the best way to lose weight before my wedding or after having one of my children. I didn't look at food as fuel (which is what I believe God intends it to be). God didn't give the Israelites dessert out in the desert; He gave them manna and quail. While I have no issue with an occasional treat, I believe we need to take a closer look at our relationship with food. And while I am far from perfect, the food I eat now is delicious and beneficial to my health most of the time. When I choose to indulge, I know I can get right back on track with the very next meal.

Another consideration when it comes to diet is bio-individuality. What works for one person may not work well for someone else. I recommend experimenting with foods and paying attention to how you feel after you eat. Keeping a food journal for a few days can provide valuable insight into how food is impacting you.

Why is a whole-foods diet necessary and beneficial to the mind, body, and spirit?

- It provides nutrient density with essential vitamins, minerals, and omega-3 fatty acids.
- It offers high-quality protein for muscle maintenance, satiety, and weight management.
- It supports heart health with healthy fats, omega-3s, and antioxidants.
- It promotes hormonal balance with essential fats and phytonutrients.
- It enhances digestive health with dietary fiber and probiotics.
- It boosts immune support with zinc, selenium, vitamins, and antioxidants.
- It reduces inflammation with anti-inflammatory properties and antioxidants.
- It strengthens bone health with calcium, vitamin D, magnesium, and phosphorus.
- It supports cognitive function with healthy fats, B vitamins, and antioxidants.

Tip

Start slowly here. If you are primarily eating a Standard American Diet (SAD), begin by cutting out processed foods. If you are eating out for lunch every day, cut back and start packing your lunch. I like to make extra servings at dinner so there is enough for lunch the next day. You could also start doing some meal prepping.

I'm a believer in organic food. If you can't afford to switch completely to organic, you can review the Clean Fifteen and Dirty Dozen at EWG.org.

Small, consistent steps are what matter most. At the end of the day, we are all bio-individuals, and no one way of eating is best for everyone. It may take some experimenting to see which foods work best for your body. All will benefit from a reduction in processed foods (especially sugar and seed oils).

Prayer

Holy Spirit, please forgive me for the times when I have indulged in food and drink that do not build up Your temple. I know it is OK to have an occasional treat, but moderation is definitely the key. Forgive me when I slip up and enable me to get right back on track. Thanks for never giving up on me. I'm so grateful for Your patience.

Reflection

What one thing can I start today that will improve what I am putting into my temple? Cut back or cut out sugar? Start packing leftovers for lunch?

....

....

....

....

....

....

....

....

....

....

Action Step

Look up the Clean Fifteen and Dirty Dozen on the EWG website and start implementing the lists. Cut out sweets this week and see how you feel.

The food you eat can either be the safest
and most powerful form of medicine,
or the slowest form of poison.
—Ann Wigmore

Clean Water

For years I struggled with symptoms of dehydration: fuzzy thinking, fatigue, headaches, joint pain, and even constipation. I had no idea that I simply needed to drink more water and cut back a bit on things like alcohol and caffeine that further dehydrate. I also had to get past the idea that I needed something more "flavorful" and fun to drink.

The rule of thumb in the functional medicine world is that you drink one-half your body weight in ounces per day. I would add that electrolyte products can be beneficial for some (especially if you are using distilled water). The color of your urine is a good indicator on hydration. If your toilet water is pale yellow or clear after you urinate, your hydration is probably on point. Dark yellow or amber colored urine are signs that your body needs fluids. When in doubt, head for the spout!

Why is proper hydration necessary and beneficial to the mind, body, and spirit?

- It promotes saliva production for oral health and food breakdown.
- It regulates body temperature and prevents overheating.
- It protects tissues, the spinal cord, and joints by providing lubrication.
- It aids in waste excretion through perspiration, urination, and bowel movements.
- It maximizes physical performance by preventing dehydration.
- It prevents constipation with adequate hydration and fiber.
- It aids digestion and enhances nutrient absorption.

- It improves blood oxygen circulation and cell communication.
- It boosts energy levels by activating metabolism.
- It enhances cognitive function, focus, and memory.
- It improves mood and reduces fatigue and anxiety.
- It keeps the skin hydrated and may support collagen production.
- It prevents overall dehydration and related complications.
- It supports brain health by enhancing neuroplasticity, facilitating nutrient transport, promoting efficient energy usage, aiding detoxification, ensuring smooth neuronal communication, and supporting cognitive functions like learning and memory.

Tip

My number one tip regarding hydration is to place a glass of water on your nightstand at bedtime. The first thing you should do when you wake up is to drink that water and replace the fluids you lost while you slept.

Clean water is especially important as our water supply (especially tap) is full of toxins. Well water can also have bacteria, chemicals, and metals. I recommend filtering and testing your water. For more information on tap quality see www.clearlyfiltered.com and for well water see www.mytapscore.com.

Prayer

Giver of all good gifts, thank You for the incredible resource of water. Without it I would die within days! Help me to prioritize drinking it over other "more flavorful" alternatives as it has so many roles in keeping the body running its best.

Reflection

Am I prioritizing hydration? How can I make drinking water easier? Do I need to cut back on or cut out dehydrating drinks?

....
....
....
....
....
....
....

Action Step

Start placing a glass of water near you at bedtime. Be sure to drink it first thing when you wake up. Test your water whether it is tap or well.

Water is the only drink for a wise man.
—Henry David Thoreau

Clean Air

I often emphasize the importance of the big three when I start working with clients. Clean food, clean water, and clean air. I learned this lesson the hard way as I ended up getting sick from mold exposure when we moved into our newly renovated 1940s farmhouse in the spring of 2020. The one area that wasn't renovated was the old basement (the source of the mold that was circulating in the air). That mold, along with all the off gassing from the new building materials and furniture and an ineffective HVAC system, was too much for my body to contend with. Thank goodness I was able to safely remediate the mold, update the HVAC system, and purchase high-quality air filters to help me recover.

Why is clean air necessary and beneficial to the mind, body, and spirit?

- Clean air boosts happiness by increasing oxygen levels and serotonin release.
- It cleanses the lungs by improving oxygen exchange and reducing pollutants.
- It strengthens the immune system by supporting oxygen supply and toxin elimination.
- It improves the digestive system by enhancing oxygen flow and circulation.
- It reduces airborne illnesses and infections by promoting ventilation and cleanliness.
- It increases energy and sharpens the mind by boosting brain function and productivity.
- It enhances sleep quality by promoting relaxation through increased serotonin.

- It prolongs lifespan by improving overall health and reducing risks associated with poor air quality.

Tip

I recommend using air filters in your home to address any airborne toxins. Depending on the air quality in your area, I also recommend getting out into fresh air and opening windows as much as you can.

Prayer

Father, forgive us for polluting the water, food, and air with man-made toxins that impact your world and our health. Help us to be better stewards of your world. Thank You for modern inventions like water and air filters that can help us avoid the negative impacts of pollution on our health.

Reflection

Do I have access to fresh air? Are there possible toxins in my home that could require an air filter?

....
....
....
....
....
....
....

Action Step

Research air filters to help address any airborne toxins in your home.

> Of all the remedies I have used or seen in use, I can find but one thing that I can call remedial for the whole disease ... and that is a profuse supply of fresh air.
>
> —Florence Nightingale

EPILOGUE

I recently took a trip to Europe. What a blessing to be able to explore new counties and cultures. About two-thirds of the way through the trip, we ran into a minor travel glitch with our train from Amsterdam to Brussels. While my husband remained quite calm, I did not. Once plans got back on track, I reflected on how upset I had gotten and how dysregulated my nervous system had become. I realized that I had neglected many of these practices throughout the trip. I was not getting morning sun, my sleep routine was nonexistent, and I was eating more sugar and drinking more alcohol than I normally would. While I was getting a lot of steps in, I missed my weight sessions. I decided to commit to prioritizing the practices from this devotion for the remainder of the trip.

I forced a smile as I lugged my suitcase up the many steps outside the Royal Library of Belgium. I silently prayed and thanked God that we were able to find an alternate route when our train from Amsterdam to Brussels was canceled. I took a bath shortly after I arrived in the room. I complimented my server at dinner and hopefully brightened his day. The next morning, I got out into the sunlight first thing and worked out in the tiny fitness center at my hotel. I nourished my body with a protein-rich breakfast and carved out some time to read my devotion. Little by little, one practice after the other helped to regulate my nervous system and calmed my demeanor.

I'm reminded time and time again how important slowing down and prioritizing these practices are to my overall health and well-being. My hope is that this devotional is one you will use over and over and that we may all find the grace to prioritize our well-being, no matter the circumstances.

ABOUT THE AUTHOR

PATRICIA MCNAMARA is a nutritional therapy practitioner, a master restorative wellness practition-er, certified midlife coach, and Neurofit certified trainer. She enjoys spending quality time with her husband and adult children while educating others about the benefits of proper nutrition and lifestyle. Her expertise focuses on supporting midlife women and nervous system regulation.

INFORMATION RESOURCES

Rest and Self Care

Cherry, Heather. "The Benefits of Resting and How to Unplug in a Busy World." Last modified December 10, 2021, at 09:42am (EST). https://www.forbes.com/sites/womensmedia/2021/01/15/the-benefits-of-resting-and-how-to-unplug-in-a-busy-world/.

Wiginton, Keri. "What Happens to your Body When you Relax." Last modified August 29, 2024, at https://www.webmd.com/balance/ss/slideshow-what-happens-when-relax.

Movement/Exercise

Champion, Chayil. "No Pain, No Gain? Training Too Hard can have Serious Health Consequences." UCLA Health. Effective November 17, 2023. https://www.uclahealth.org/news/article/no-pain-no-gain-training-too-hard-can-have-serious-Health.

NIH National Institute on Aging (NIA). "Real-Life Benefits of Exercise and Physical Activity." Last modified April 3, 2020, at https://www.nia.nih.gov/health/exercise-and-physical-activity/real-life-benefits-exercise-and-Physical-activity/.

Morning Sunlight

Isabel, Cody. "The Neuroscience behind Sunlight's Benefits: A Ray of Hope for Mental Health." The Mind, Brain, Body Digest. Effective March 30, 2023. https://blog.mindbrainbodylab.com/p/the-neuroscience-behind-sunlights.

Nazish, Noma. "Why Sunlight Is Actually Good For You." Last modified June 28, 2021, at 10:57am (EDT). https://www.forbes.com/sites/nomanazish/2018/02/28/why-sunlight-is-actually-good-for-you/.

Sleep

National Cancer Institute. "Alcohol and Cancer Risk Fact Sheet." Cancer.gov, U.S. Department of Health and Human Services, August 1, 2023. https://www.cancer.gov/about-cancer/causes-prevention/risk/alcohol/alcohol-fact-sheet.

Summer, Jay and Abhinav Singh. "8 Health Benefits of Sleep." Last modified February 29, 2024, at https://www.sleepfoundation.org/how-sleep-works/benefits-of-sleep.

Stibich, Mark. "10 Benefits of Sleep." Last modified May 18, 2023, at https://www.verywellhealth.com/top-health-benefits-of-a-good-nights-sleep-2223766.

Mindset and Visualization

Davis, Tchiki and Kelsey Schultz. "How Visualization Can Benefit Your Well-Being." Last modified November 20, 2023, at https://www.psychologytoday.com/intl/blog/click-here-for-happiness/202308/how-visualization-can-benefit-your-well-being

Acts of Kindness

Sreenivasan, Shoba and Linda E. Weinberger. "Why Random Acts of Kindness Matter to Your Well-being." Psychology Today. Effective November 16, 2017. https://www.psychologytoday.com/us/blog/emotional-nourishment/201711/why-random-acts-kindness-matter-your-well-being#:~:text=Compassion%20and%20kindness%20also%20reduce%20stress%2C%20boost%20our,more%20likely%20to%20be%20kind%20to%20other%20people.

Gratitude

Logan, Amnanda. "Can Expressing Gratitude Improve your Mental, Physical Health?" Mayo Clinic Health System. Effective December 6, 2022. https://www.mayoclinichealthsystem.org/hometown-health/speaking-of-health/can-expressing-gratitude-improve-health#:~:text=Expressing%20gratitude%20is%20associated%20with%20a%20host%20of,could%20do%20this%2C%20everyone%20would%20be%20taking%20it.

Miller, Kori D. "14 Benefits of Practicing Gratitude (Incl. Journaling)." Positive Psychology. Effective June 18, 2019. https://positivepsychology.com/benefits-of-gratitude/.

Prayer

Vann, Madeline R., and Sarah Garone. "Is Prayer Good for Your Health?" Everyday Health. Last modified October 5, 2023, at https://www.everydayhealth.com/emotional-health/power-of-prayer.aspx

Journaling

Bennett, Kevin. "10 Good Reasons to Keep a Journal." Psychology Today. Last modified January 31, 2023, at https://www.psychologytoday.com/us/blog/modern-minds/202301/10-good-reasons-to-keep-a-journal

Play

Harvard Medical School. "Dancing and the brain." Accessed October 4, 2024. https://hms.harvard.edu/news-events/publications-archive/brain/dancing-brain.

Robinson, Lawrence, Melinda Smith, Jeanne Segal, and Jennifer Shubin. "The Benefits of Play for Adults." HelpGuide.org. Last modified June 4, 2024, at https://www.helpguide.org/articles/mental-health/benefits-of-play-for-adults.htm.

Nature and Grounding

Gregory, Sara Youngblood. "The Mental Health Benefits of Nature: Spending Time Outdoors to Refresh Your Mind." Mayo Clinic. Effective March 4, 2024. https://mcpress.mayoclinic.org/mental-health/the-mental-health-benefits-of-nature-spending-time-outdoors-to-refresh-your-mind/.

Breathwork

Cleveland Clinic. "Breathwork for Beginners: What to Know and How to Get Started." Cleveland Clinic. Effective May 19, 2023. https://health.clevelandclinic.org/breathwork.

Othership. "15 Breathwork Benefits: The Science behind Breathing Practices." Othership. Effective August 19, 2021. https://www.othership.us/resources/breathwork-benefits

Staying Present

Perry, Elizabeth. "Here and Now: Discover the Benefits of Being Present." Better Up. Effective March 10, 2022. https://www.betterup.com/blog/how-to-be-present#:~:text=Present%20moment%20awareness%20over%20time,knowledge%20and%20improve%20our%20skills.

Yoga (Sacred Stretch)

John Hopkins Medicine. "9 Benefits of Yoga." Accessed October 3, 2024. https://www.hopkinsmedicine.org/health/wellness-and-prevention/9-benefits-of-yoga/

Contentment

American Heart Association. "How Happiness Affects Health." Last reviewed May 20, 2020. https://www.heart.org/en/university-hospitals-.

Good Therapy. "The Good Therapy Blog." Accessed October 3, 2024. https://www.goodtherapy.org/blog/the-essence-of-contentment-how-acceptance-promotes-Happiness-0911194

Sutton, Jeremy. "5+ Benefits of Positive Emotions on Psychological Wellbeing." Positive Psychology. Effective December 13, 2016. https://positivepsychology.com/benefits-of-positive-emotions/.

Boundaries

Oswald, Rich. "Map It Out: Setting Boundaries for Your Well-being." Mayo Clinic Health System. Effective December 27, 2023. https://www.mayoclinichealthsystem.org/hometown-health/speaking-of-health/setting-Boundaries-for-well-being.

Laughter

Mayo Clinic Staff. "Healthy Lifestyle: Stress Management." Mayo Clinic. Effective September 22, 2023. https://www.mayoclinic.org/healthy-lifestyle/stress-management/in-depth/stress-relief/art-20044456.

Community

Stein, Samantha. "The Importance of Community." Psychology Today. Effective July 18, 2023. https://www.psychologytoday.com/us/blog/what-the-wild-things-are/202307/the-importance-of-community

Digital Detox

Sreenivas, Shishira. "Digital Detox: What to Know." WebMD. Effective May 5, 2023. https://www.webmd.com/balance/what-is-digital-detox.

Christian Meditation

Aura Meditation Guide. "Exploring the Benefits of Christian Meditation and Mindfulness." Aura Health. Effective June 7, 2023. https://www.aurahealth.io/blog/christian-meditation-and-

mindfulness#:~:text=One%20of%20the%20most%20
significant,sense%20of%20purpose%20and%20fulfillment.

Nourishment

Axe, Josh. "Top Nutrient-Dense Foods and Their Benefits." Dr.
Axe. Effective September 26, 2021. https://draxe.com/nutrition/
nutrient-dense-foods/.

Bendix, Aria. "11 Terrifying Things That Could Be Lurking In Your
Tap Water." Business Insider. Effective July 5, 2019. https://www.
businessinsider.com/toxic-chemicals-tap-drinking-water-2019-
4#radioactive-substances-can-leech-into-groundwater-which-has-
become-a-huge-problem-in-texas-3.

Blackwood, Michelle. "Fresh Air Benefits." Healthier Steps. Effective
July 30, 2022. https://healthiersteps.com/fresh-air-benefits/.

Cleveland Clinic. "Seed Oils: Are They Actually Toxic?"
Cleveland Clinic. Effective October 4, 2023. https://health.
clevelandclinic.org/seed-oils-are-they-actually-toxic.

Huang, Yin, Zeyu Chen, Bo Chen, et al. "Dietary Sugar
Consumption and Health: Umbrella Review." *BMJ* 381 (2023):
e071609. https://doi.org/10.1136/bmj-2022-071609.

Joseph, Michael. "14 Nutrient-Dense Foods to Consider." Last
modified October 4, 2024, at https://www.nutritionadvance.
com/most-nutrient-dense-foods-in-the-world/.

Link, Rachael. "Salmon Nutrition: Wild-Caught Salmon Protects
the Brain, Bones, Eyes, Skin & More." Dr. Axe. Effective April

29, 2024. https://draxe.com/nutrition/8-salmon-nutrition-facts-proven-health-benefits/.

Mayo Clinic Staff. "Healthy Lifestyle: Nutrition and Aging." Mayo Clinic. Effective April 22, 2022. https://www.mayoclinic.org/healthy-lifestyle/nutrition-and-healthy-eating/in-depth/organic-food/art-20043880.

Paleo On The GO. "Paleo Diet: Get Fiber from Real, Whole Foods." Accessed October 3, 2024. https://paleoonthego.com/blogs/foods/get-fiber-from-paleo.

Sacred Cow. "About the Film." Accessed October 3, 2024. https://www.sacredcow.info/about-the-film.

Silver, Natalie. "Why Is Water Important? 16 Reasons to Drink Up." Last modified April 12, 2023, at https://www.healthline.com/health/food-nutrition/why-is-water-important.

Very Big Brain. "Water Intake and Neuroplasticity: The Hydration-Brain Link." Very Big Brain. Effective November 21, 2023. https://verybigbrain.com/body-brain-connection/water-intake-and-neuroplasticity-the-hydration-brain-link/.

Wolf, Robb. "Why is Hydration Important? (10 Benefits of Staying Hydrated)." Accessed October 3, 2024. https://science.drinklmnt.com/did-you-know/10-benefits-of-staying-hydrated/.

Printed in the United States
by Baker & Taylor Publisher Services